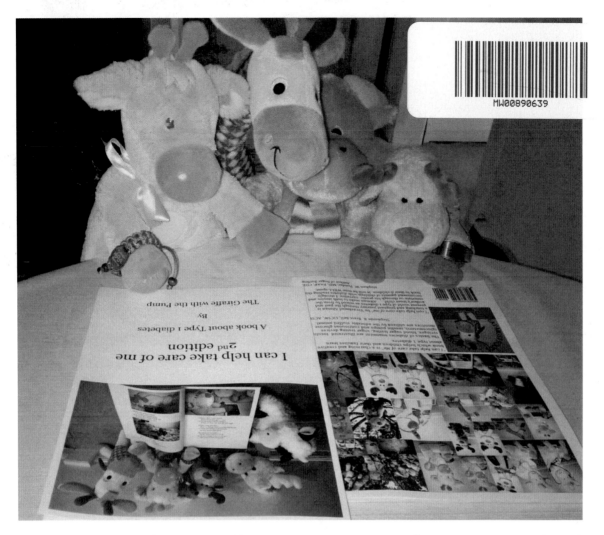

I can help take care of me 2nd edition

A book about Type 1 diabetes

By

The Giraffe with the Pump

© 2018 Yerachmiel Altman

All rights reserved. No portion of this book may be reproduced in any form without permission from the author, except as permitted by U.S. copyright law.

For permissions contact: YBA613@hotmail.com

ISBN-13: 978-1530374892

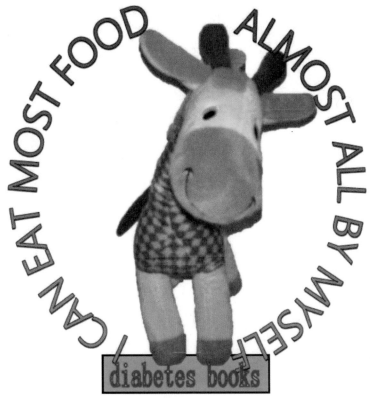

I CAN EAT MOST FOOD ALMOST ALL BY MYSELF

diabetes books

I've had diabetes
   Since I was just two.
The outlook was much different then:
   Tools and testing too.

Syringes made of glass,
   Boiled to sterilize.
Couldn't test blood sugar,
   So Clinitest we tried

I got my first pump
   When they were brand new.
Bigger and more trouble and
   One basal rate, it's true.

But now there's great equipment
   And medical staff who cares.
We have to learn the rules
   Which in this book I'll share.

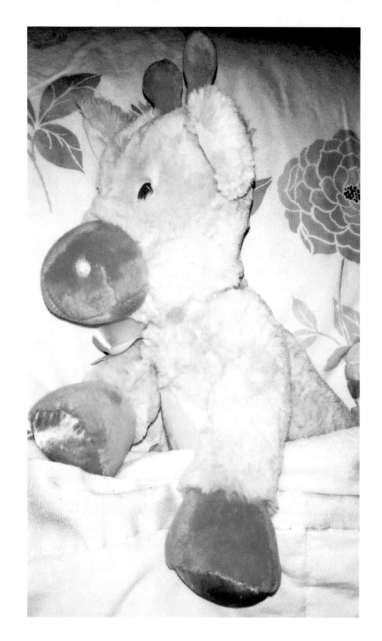

One day I felt quite strange,
  Yucky, slow and sick.
Way too tired to walk,
  Couldn't move so quick.

My head and tummy hurt,
  I wanted to drink and drink.
So knocked out and weak,
  Didn't know what to think.

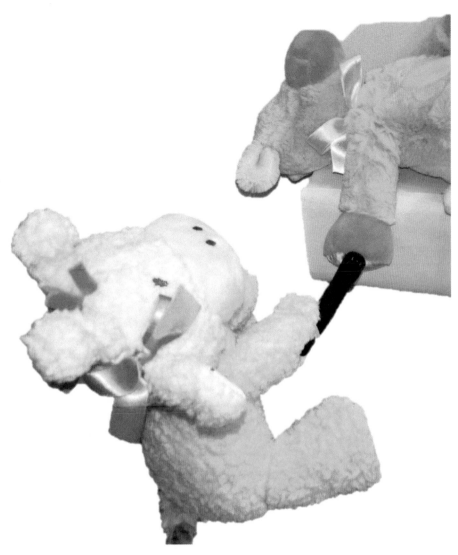

Mom took me to the doc
    Because I felt like mud.
He checked eyes and ears,
    And said he'd check my blood.

With a strip in a machine,
    And a needle in a pen.
The pen touched my finger,
    He pressed a button, then...

A drop of blood came out
    He touched it to that stick
The machine began to count
    It finished and beeped quick!

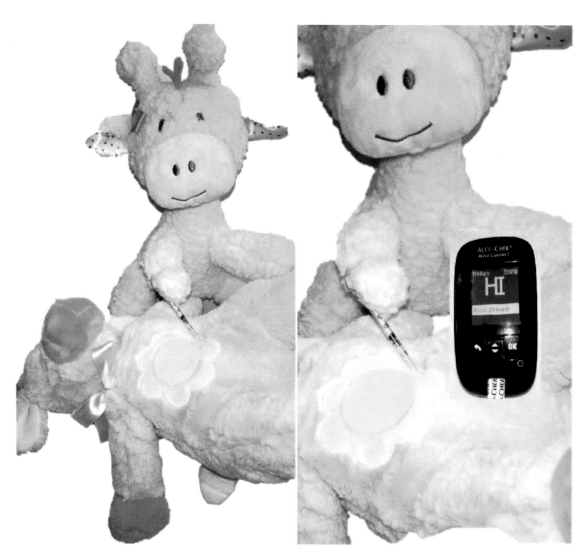

Doctor said "The meter
　　Reads the sugar in your blood
HI means so much there
　　It's sort of like a flood

With special medication
　　In a needle you'll learn to take
You'll begin to feel much better,
　　You'll play, smile and not ache!

Because the machine says "HI"
　　You right away will take
Things for a short visit,
　　To the hospital you will make

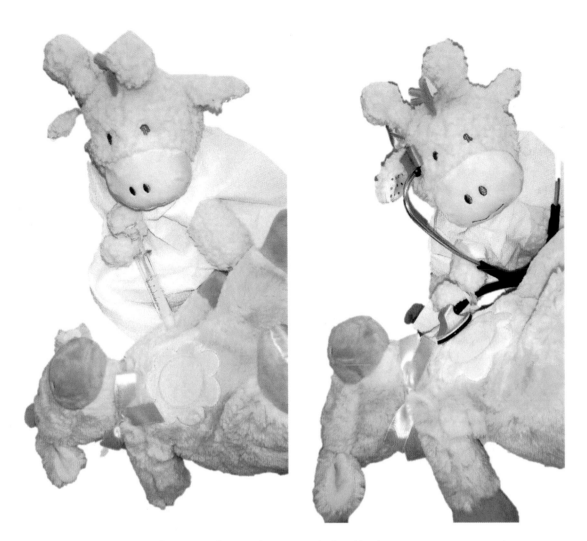

When the doc said diabetes
  Was the illness that I had
I didn't know what it was
  But I knew I was not glad

I didn't know what it meant
  Or why all those blood tests
And why so many shots
  That I never got to rest

Type One Diabetes
  Was what they said I had
But I did nothing wrong
  And I wasn't bad

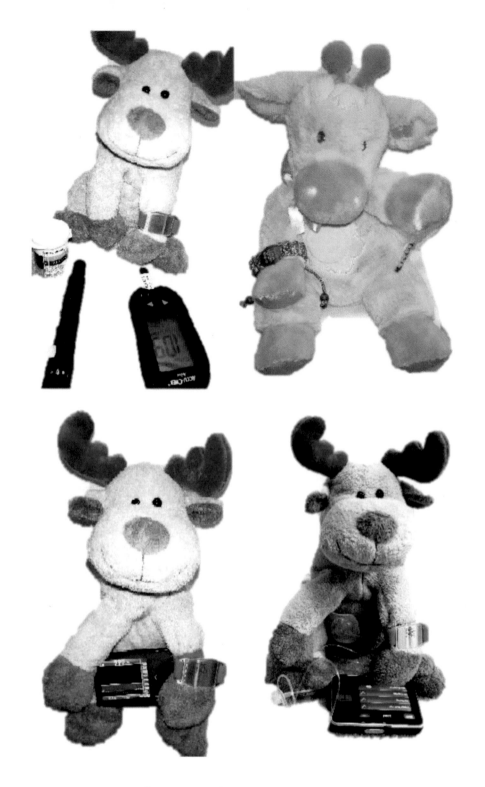

I would now learn
    how to take good care
Take a shot, wear a pump
    Test my blood anywhere

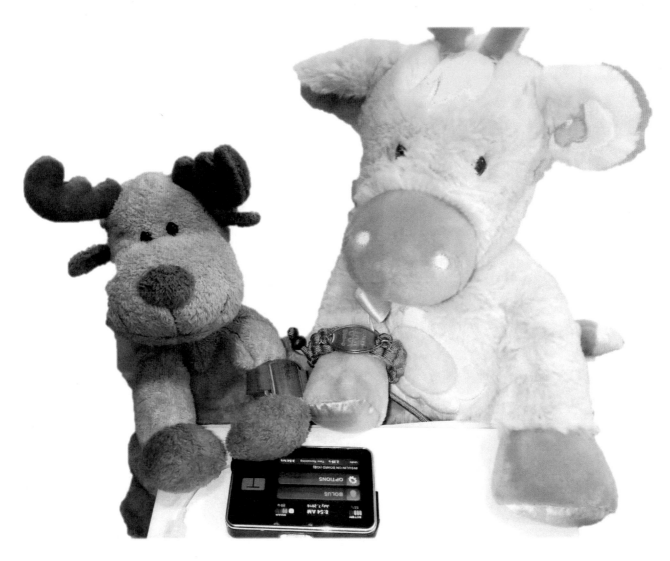

I know that I can teach
    Important things to you.
Your parents will be happy
    When at last we're through.

Tricky they are not;
    They're things that you should know
To help you keep your health
    As you learn and grow.

The body is complex.
    Rules don't always work.
If sugar's out of range,
    The system has its quirks.

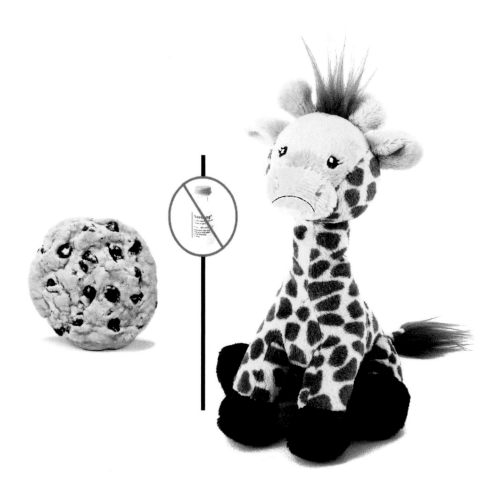

Diabetes comes,
    When the body stops
    Making insulin,
        And then you must take shots.

The body's insulin
    Acts just like a key.
Gets food into our cells
    So we have energy.

Without insulin
    One could eat day and night
But they can't use the food
    It's as though out of sight

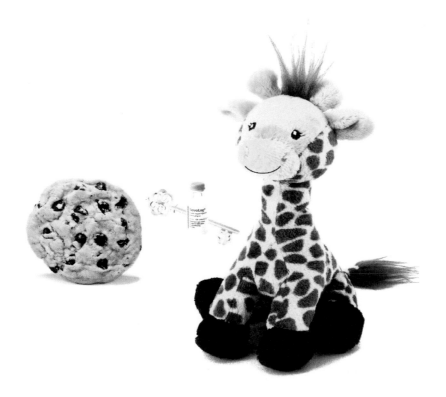

When we eat good food
   like fruit or milk or steak,
Our stomach breaks it down
   so that we can take

The energy from food
   in head and arms and feet.
Without the insulin,
   It's like we didn't eat.

Just like your own house has
   A lock upon the door,
You cannot get inside, not even
   Crawling on the floor!

But with that tiny key
   You get in and play.
Insulin's the same,
   Frees up energy all day.

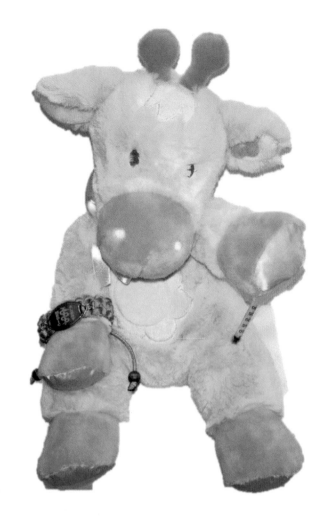

Quickly I did learn
   To take an insulin shot!
I did it by myself
   Easy, it was not.

But now I fill my dose
   And check it has no air.
I must take it when
   There are no bubbles there.

A needle I can give
   In leg or arm or tum,
And sometimes even I
   Can give it in my bum.

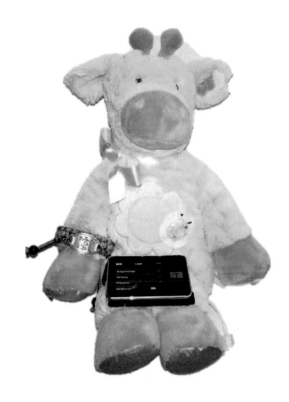

Then I got a pump
   Which holds my insulin.
Instead of taking shots
   I keep a needle in.

With my handy pump
   I bolus the right dose.
For food it is much easier
   I don't need needles close.

Either way will work
   And while they are not fun
They'll help me stay in range
   As well as can be done.

I always try my best
And ask if I'm not sure.
I know I'll need my insulin
   Until there is a cure.

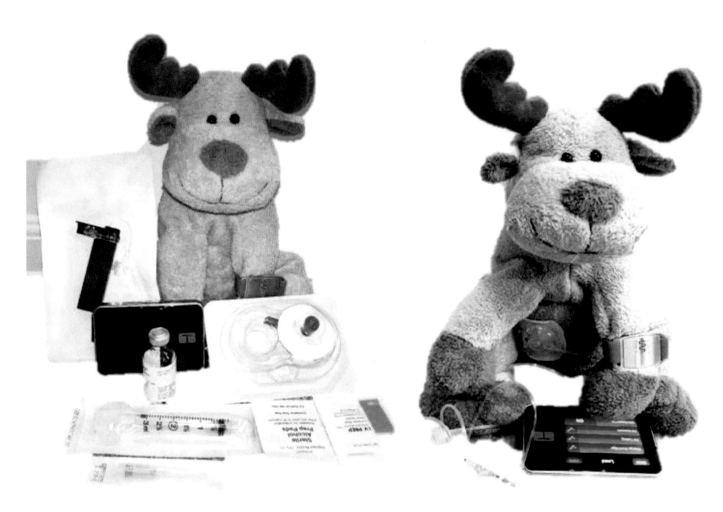

My pump has insulin
   Which day and night it gives.
And when I want to eat,
   A bolus helps me live.

The pump must be refilled
   Every couple of days.
And also a new set,
   Which I put in; it stays!

I have to charge my pump
   To make sure it has power,
Some pumps get batteries,
   And others charge by hour.

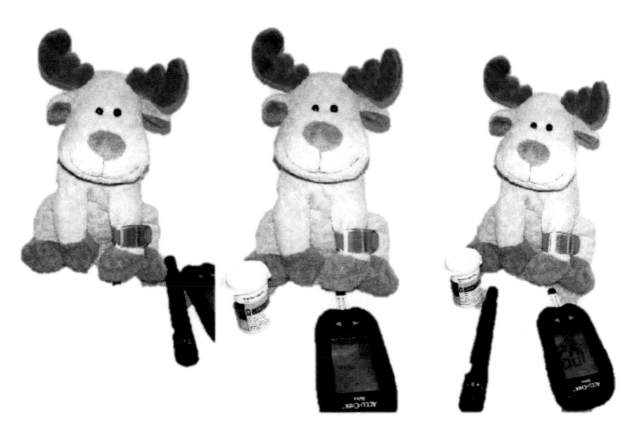

This, my glucose meter,
   Blood sugar it does see.
I take blood from my finger,
   My arm, but not my knee.

A blood test I must take
   Several times a day
To see just how I'm doing
   so I can freely play.

I put the test strip in
   The meter that I use.
The lancet will take blood,
   From the finger that I choose.

The drop goes on the strip.
   The meter starts to count.
Then it will display
   My sugar's right amount.

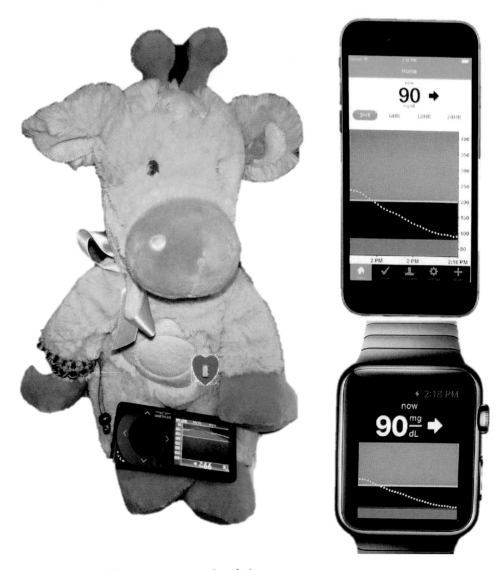

My sensor's like a meter
  To keep track of my reading.
So that I can tell
  When I should be eating.

It takes my readings often,
  And it lets me know
If my sugar's high
  Or if it is too low.

The readings it can show
  or send them through a phone.
My parents won't be worried
  When I am out alone.

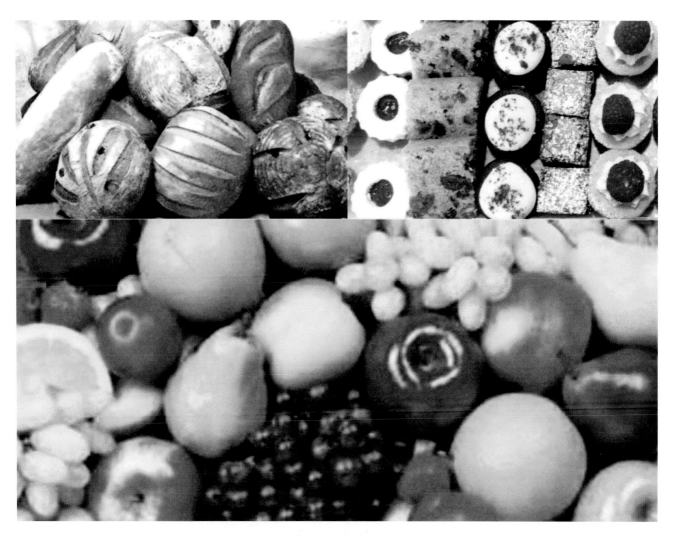

Carbohydrates are
    Our source of energy.
To sugar they will turn and then
    We'll use them properly.

The insulin we need
    To allow the food to work.
It keeps us all alive,
    And never does it shirk.

We would really like
    Diabetes to go away, but
Until it's figured out, our shots
    Of insulin will stay.

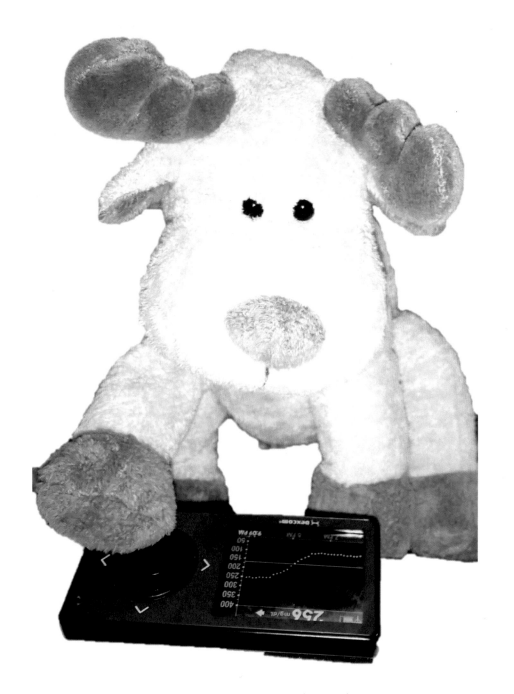

Your meter says No! No!
    You cannot go; just stay!
It says that you will need
    Correcting before play.

When blood sugar's low
    Or when it is too high,
It says you must correct
    And now I'll tell you why.

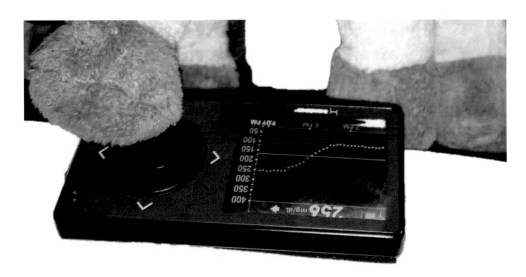

When my sugar's high
   I really want to sleep,
I get all tired out
   And to my bed I creep.

The bathroom I might need,
   And I feel really sick.
I drink a lot of water,
   And my head feels thick.

Then I do my test,
   To find out just how high.
I maybe ate too much,
   Or my shot was shy.

Could be my set came out,
   But in any case
I will need a shot.
   It will not leave a trace.

I listen to my folks
   And do as doc would say.
I think it is not fun
   But I will be okay.

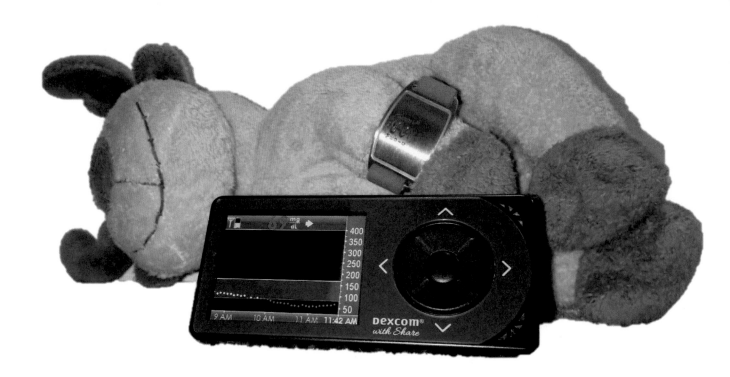

When my sugar's low,
   Immediately I'll eat.
If I'm not careful, then
   I might fall off my feet.

It means no energy
   To run or play or think.
It must be treated NOW,
   So further it won't sink.

I need somebody's help
   To bring me juice and QUICK!
Or give me glucagon,
   So I won't get real sick.

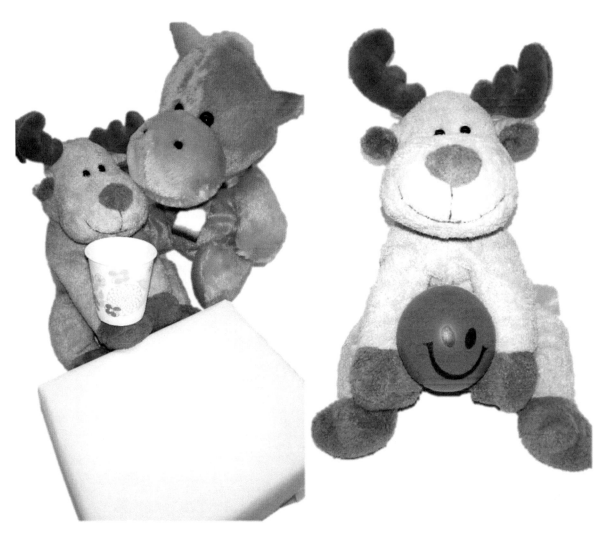

A simple glass of juice.
　　Again, I feel OK.
But I have to wait
　　Until I'm fit to play.

After a short time,
　　I'm back out with my friends.
Our fun will start again because
　　Low sugar quickly mends!

Remembering this time
　　I'll think what I can do
Have a snack before I play
　　To make reactions few.

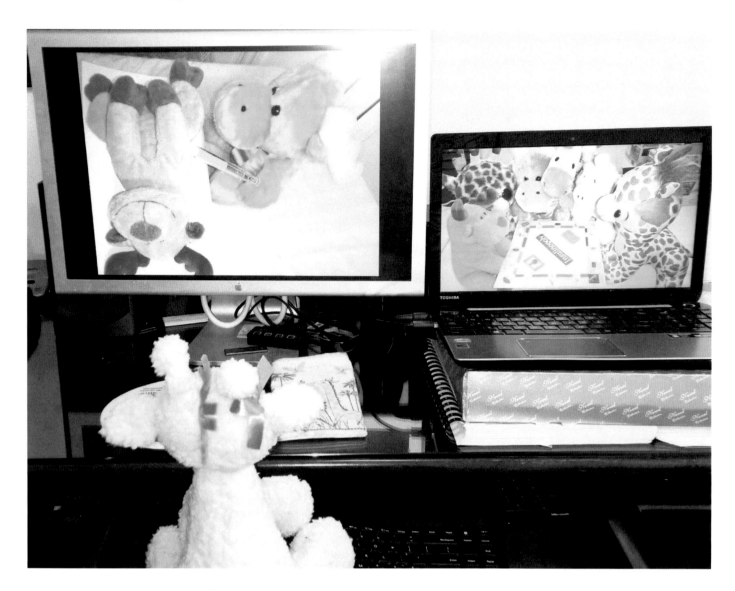

Even when I sit
   And read a funny book
Or homework, oh so hard,
   The computer needs a look.

I must always keep in mind
   That my sugar level may dip
And it's real important to treat

In fact, yes, even when
   I'm fast asleep in bed
Blood glucose can drop
   And then I must be fed.

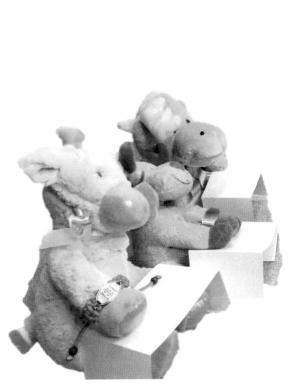
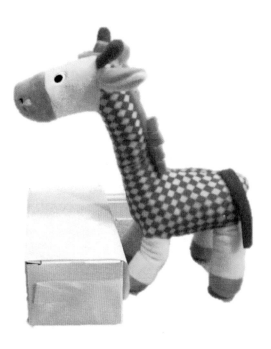

Now that I am big
   I go to school each day,
Sometimes I need a snack
   And must have it right away.

If I feel low or cold,
   Weak or tired or sick,
I have to check my sugar
   And I must do it quick.

If my sugar's high,
   Then I will correct
With some insulin
   Which I will inject.

Or if my sugar's low
   I might not know or say
That I need a snack
   To help me run and play.

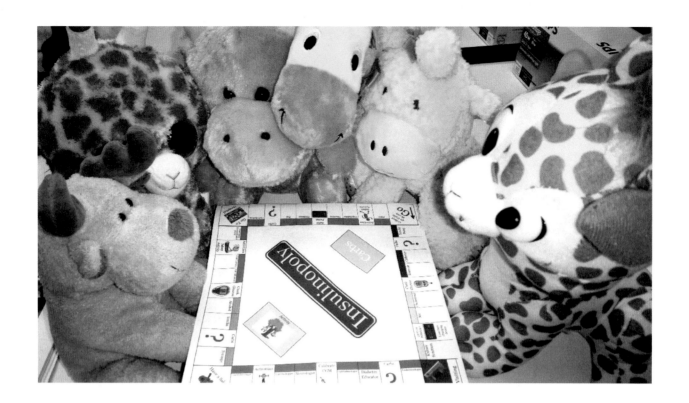

I just want my friends
    To come and truly see
I'm really just like them
    Because we all can be

In need of special help
    With things we cannot do.
It may be things to eat,
    Or even tying shoes!

We can go to school,
    eat and talk and play,
But you will never catch
    My illness in that way.

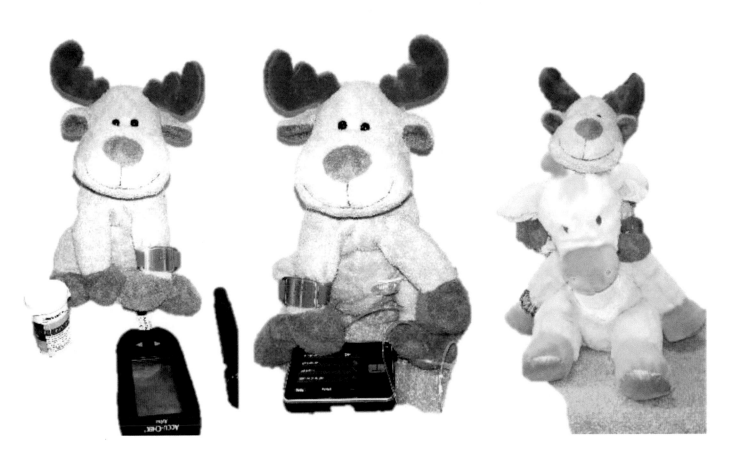

Maybe we won't eat
    exactly the same things,
But I will stay healthy
    And run and play and sing.

Friends might well be scared
    Of catching diabetes from me.
Of needing tests and shots,
    But that will never be.

They don't like it when
    Finger sticks I take,
I just ask them, please,
    To give me a short break.

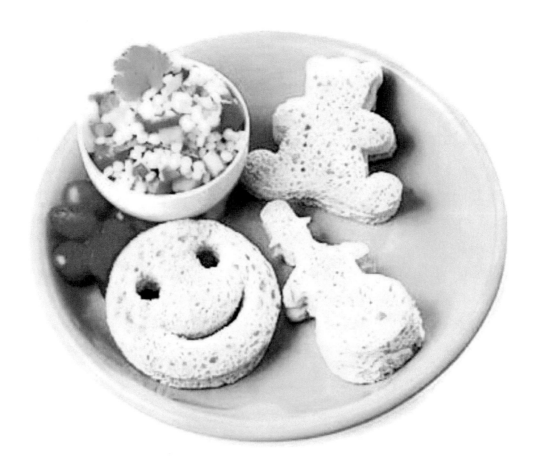

For some foods like bread,
   Or cookies or cupcakes,
It really is important
   to sum up what to take.

For some food like squash,
   Or eggs or tuna fish
You don't need insulin --
   Eat just what you wish.

If you want a drink,
   Juice, milk or iced tea
Add in all the carbs
   Unless the drink's carb free.

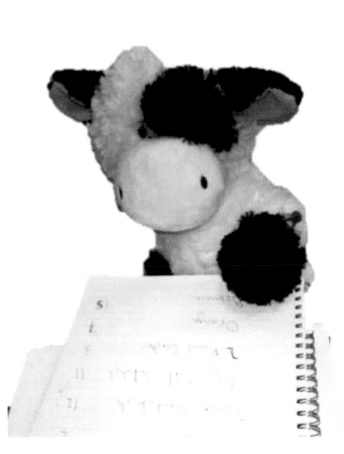

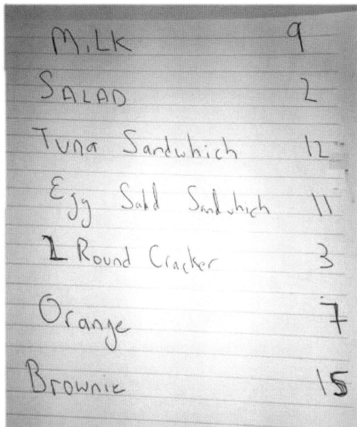

Milk — 9
Salad — 2
Tuna Sandwhich — 12
Egg Sald Sandwich — 11
1 Round Cracker — 3
Orange — 7
Brownie — 15

Insulin you need
   For each gram of carb you eat.
Take the right amount,
   And food will be a treat!

My Dad made me a book
   With the foods for when I'm out
It has the right amount to take
   For those things there is no doubt

When I go to school
   Or visit a good friend
Now it's for me to eat
   My visit won't have to end

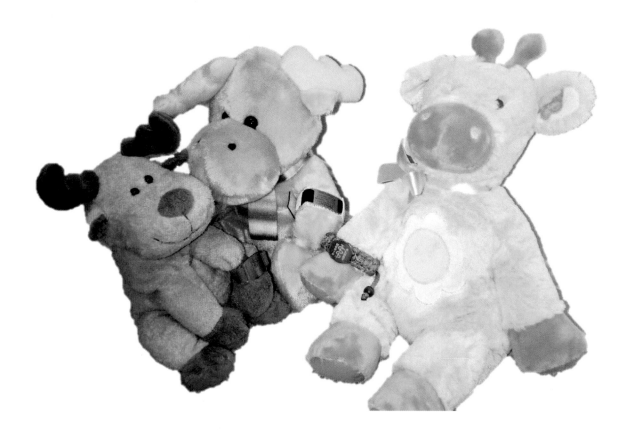

Besides my food and drink
  I've learned to live each day
With special rules and guidelines
  That I'll show you as I play

To remember I must check
  And make sure I'm OK
To always wear my Medic Alert
  To tell others if I can't say

To check my feet at night
  Put needles in their bay
To have a travel case
  For when I go away.

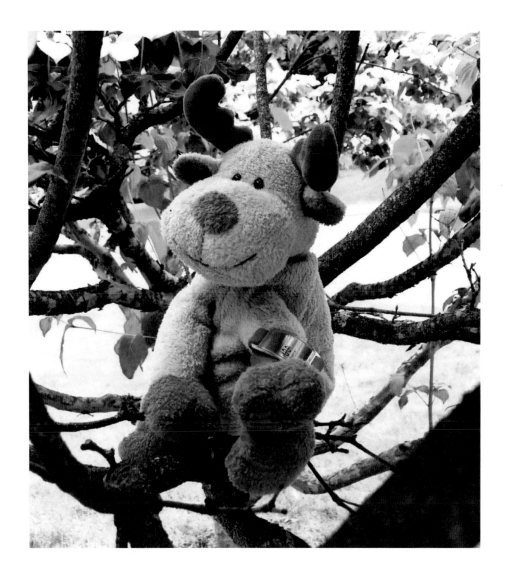

Look what's on my wrist.
　　Oh no, it doesn't hurt!
It's there if I have trouble
　　It's a medical alert!

It has information
　　On my doctor, folks and all.
If something happens to me,
　　They'll know just who to call.

I know that it's not fancy
　　Or beautiful to see,
But it could save my life.
　　I know you will agree.

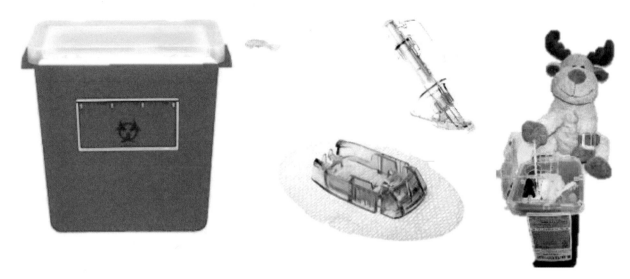

I have to be so careful.
   I must be on alert.
I must take care of needles,
   So no one will get hurt.

They should always go
   Into a special box,
Along with sets and sensors.
   We close them up with locks.

I'm careful with my test strips
   Always to be neat.
The tissue for my blood,
   I don't throw in the street.

When I want to test,
   My finger should be clean.
So I wash my hands
   No dirt can then be seen.

When I'm done, my things
   Out, I do not throw.
My special box, it is,
   The place where they will go.

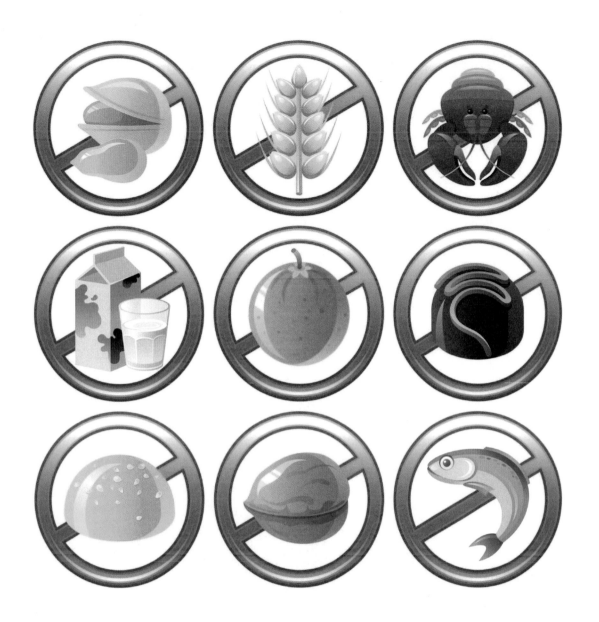

People are all different
    Some can't eat one dish.
Some cannot eat peanuts
    Or milk or bread or fish.

I have something special.
    I have a small machine.
It helps me when I eat,
    And often can't be seen.

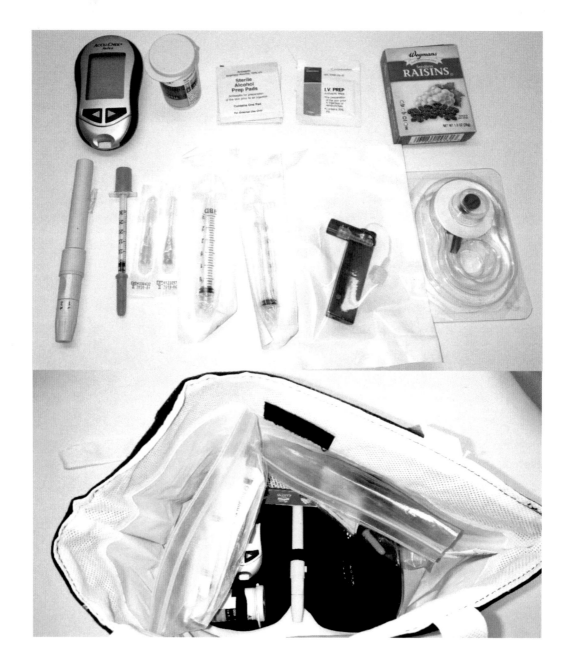

If you would like to go
   To a dear friend's house,
There is no need to fear,
   be brave; don't be a mouse.

Remember you should take
   All the things you'll need.
Following the guidelines
   Will help you to succeed.

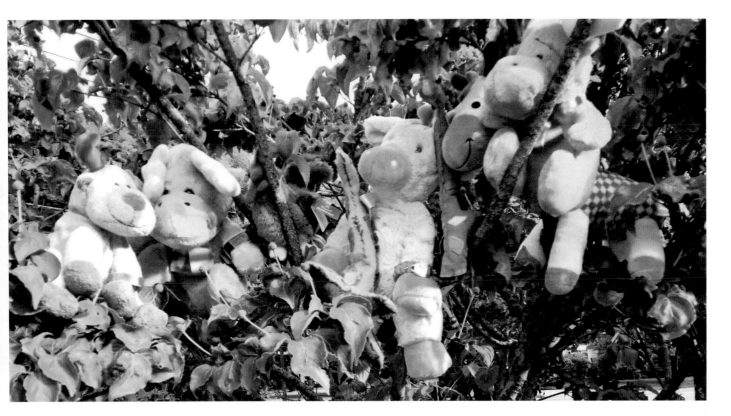

When I go and walk
　　Or swim or run so free
Or play with all my friends
　　Or climb up in a tree,

I'm careful not to let
　　My sugar ruin my fun.
So I take a snack,
　　In case I do need one!

It can be jelly beans,
　　Juice or fruit, you know.
Chocolate will not work
　　Since it is too slow.

It should be something small
　　That I can swallow well.
And if I'm acting strange
　　A friend can help me tell.

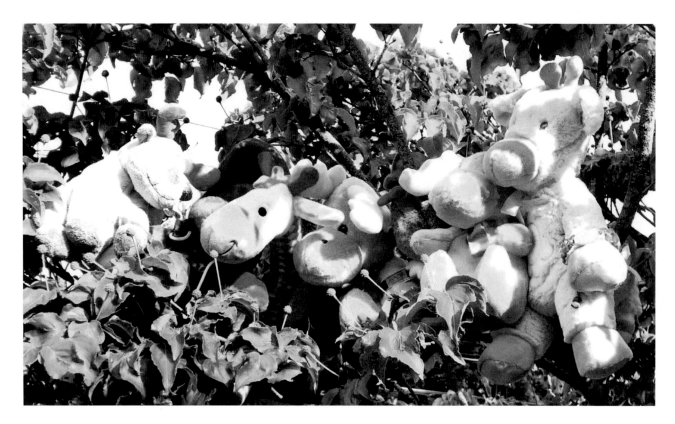

When I first found out
　　Diabetes was to blame
For making me feel sick
　　And not able to play games,

I wondered, so I asked,
　　"What will this mean to me?
Will I not be able
　　To climb up in a tree?

"Will it let me go
　　To school to learn each day,
Or let me go outside
　　With my friends to play?"

But once I learned the way
　　To take care of me
My friends and I can have fun
　　Go to school and climb a tree

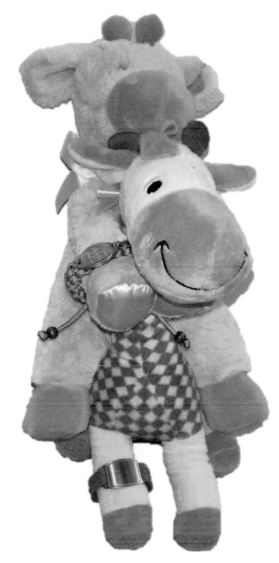

In spite of diabetes
  I can do many things.
I can dance, play and learn,
  And do chores while I sing.

I will still be careful
  and watch what I eat;
Take insulin with meals
  and with my treats.

As long as am careful
  Eating when I should
I can have fun just like my friends
  My life is very good.

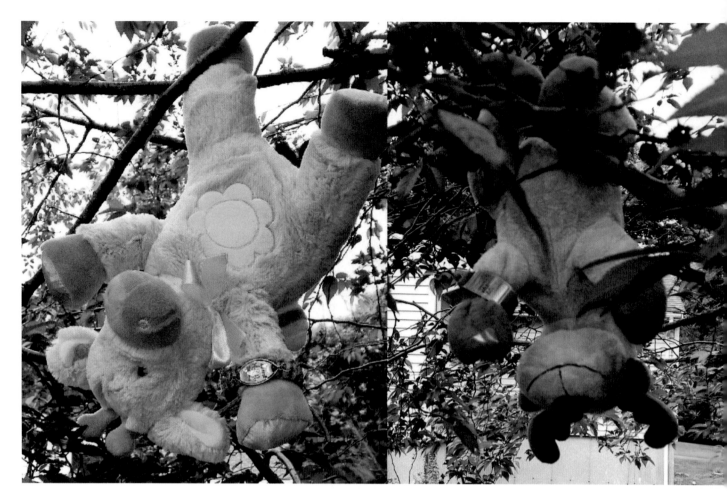

Climbing up a tree,
  Hanging upside down,
I really like to smile
  I'm happy; I don't frown.

I always watch my sugar
  Even in a tree.
I'm doing things correctly.
  My parents can trust me!

Staying healthy is important
  To having fun while at play
I'm learning about diabetes
  I get better every day

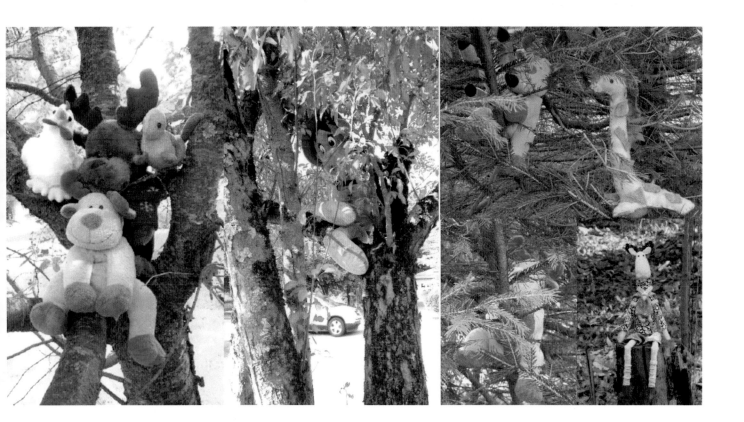

When friends come out to play,
    Or I'm out all alone,
I'm always careful with my things,
    Just like with a phone.

My pump and my sensor
    Meters, lancets and the rest
Must be kept working perfectly
    So they'll work at their best

They can't get wet or kicked,
    Or dropped or scratched or cracked
For then all of my readings
    Will be all out of whack.

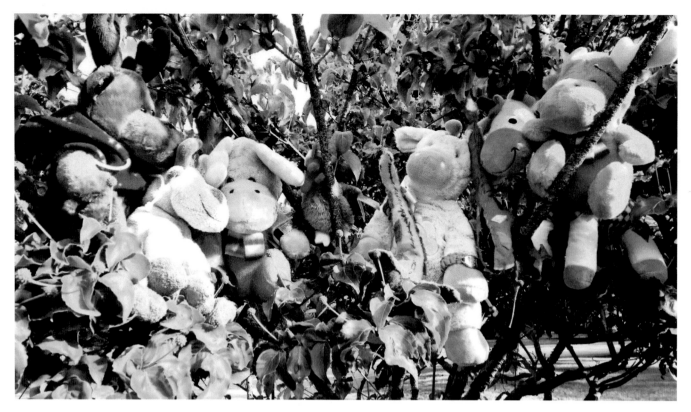

In the summer when
   I play out of doors,
I must be very careful
   That I don't get sores.

On a sunny day
   I also drink a lot,
Water is so good
   When it's very hot.

I think about the fact
   That I must sometimes eat
And not spend all the day
   Playing on my feet.

When I take a swim
   In the pool or lake.
I must protect my pump
   So it doesn't break.

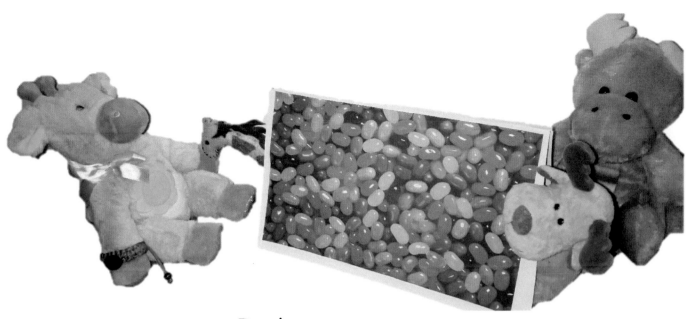

In the summer
    I go to camp Jelly Bean
Where other children
    With diabetes are seen

We live in cabins
    Like a big family
We go on camp trips
    We climb in the trees

We swim in a lake
    We make a camp fire at night
And we learn to be careful
    And we are quite a sight

When we wake up each day
    Our sugars we take
Then off to our breakfast
    And then to the lake

I love camping each summer
    With my T1 friends
We learn from each other
    If we try there's no end

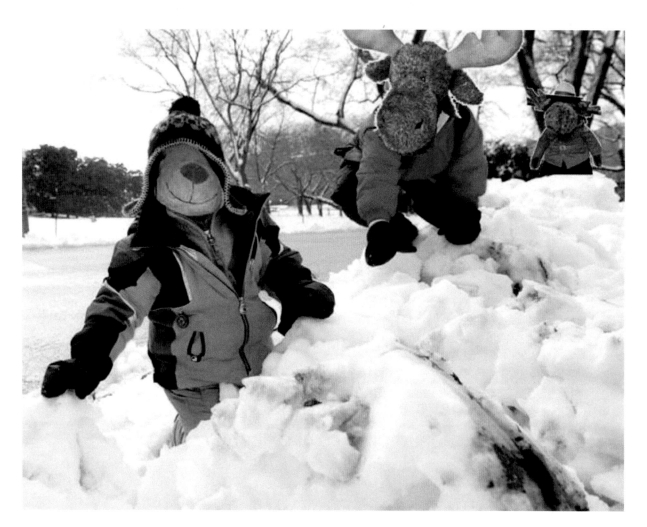

My blood sugar may fall
  When playing in snow.
But my sensor will warn me
  If it falls too low

If I'm shaky or cold
  Or find it hard to speak
Or wild and crazy
  Or tired and weak

When things don't seem normal
  It's always best to just see
If my blood sugar is off
  And to take care of me

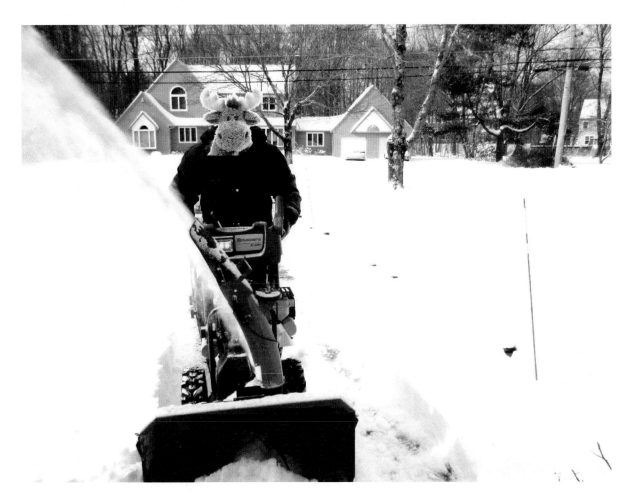

In the winter when
    it's cold outside with snow,
I have to wear my boots
    and gloves for warmth, you know.

A snowman I can make
    and angels with my friends,
As long as I snack when
    The sensor low does trend.
 Insulin is picky:
    Not too hot or cold
We must keep it safe,
    Just like we've been told.

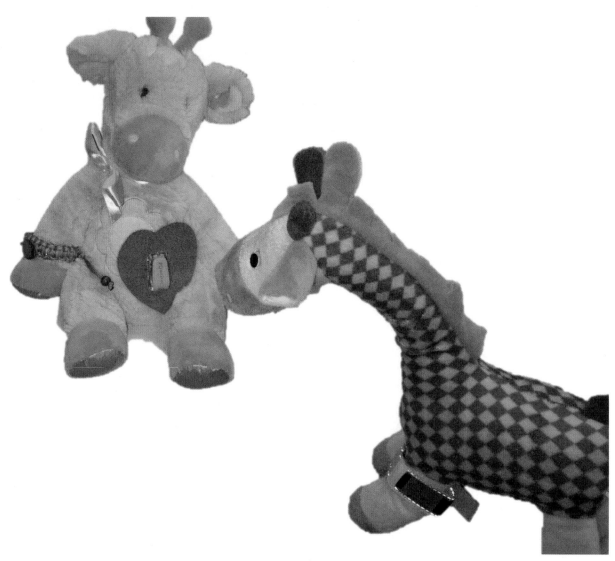

WearingDabbee helps me enjoy my sensor,
   Even on a day when I'm not keen
I put on my stickers
   And I don't mind being seen

When I check my sugar level
   On my CGM
It now has a cute cover
   Which I'm happy to show them.

They help keep it on.
   They keep it in place
I don't want to lose it.
   Dad says it's hard to replace

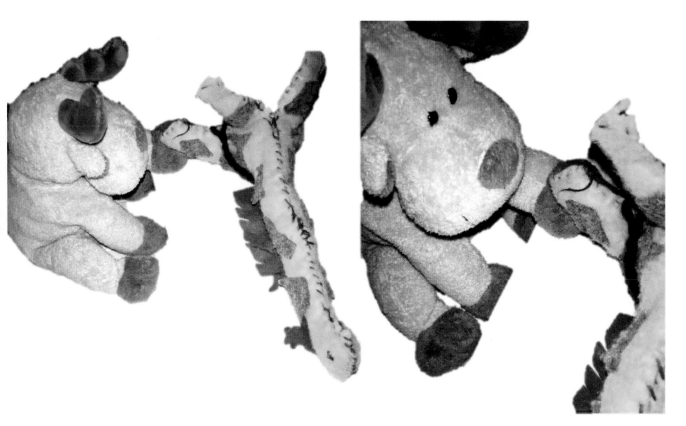

I always wear my shoes,
   Whenever I go out.
Warm slippers I'll put on
   Inside, without a doubt.

Slippers for the pool
   And for the bath they're swell,
So that both my feet
   Are taken care of well.

Every day I check
   Both my legs and feet.
To make sure there's no wounds
   And they're clean and neat.

When I play with friends,
   And fall down and get hurt,
Someone should check my wound,
   And clean off all the dirt.

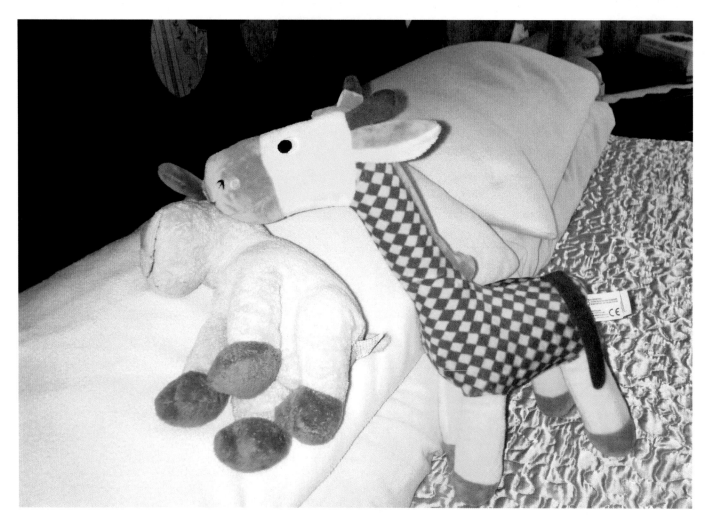

When the night has come
  To my bed I'll go.
My friends will also sleep.
  When day comes, we're not slow!

I want to keep good health
  So I must get my sleep,
Or my sugar will
  Make my sensor beep.

I'll also be too tired to
  Be careful when I must.
I might make big mistakes
  And lose my parent's trust.

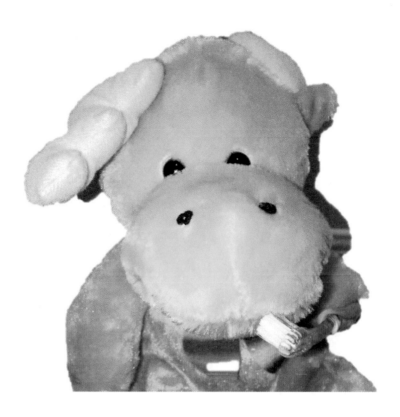

I always brush my teeth
  After food I eat,
Mommy sometimes checks
  If brushing was complete.

And when I get back home
  From school or from my play,
If I forgot, I'll brush
  So clean my teeth will stay.

I go to the dentist.
  My teeth are cleaned like new.
The dentist really likes it that
  I brush and floss them too.

He takes those funny pictures,
  By using weird cardboard,
Afterwards he looks at them
  And I get a reward.

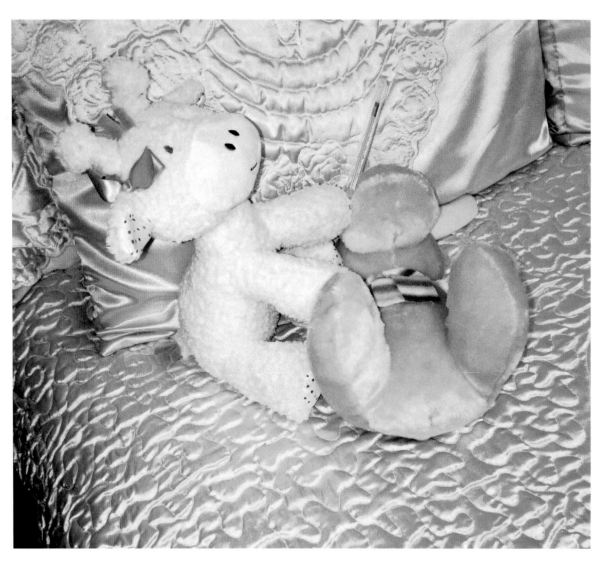

If I catch either flu or cold
  My folks know what to do.
Blood sugar must be watched
  It goes up and down, it's true.

If it starts to rise,
  A correction I will take.
It helps me to get well
  It helps to fight the ache!

If sugar starts to sink
  To fix it I arrange
By having a quick snack
  And get to healthy range

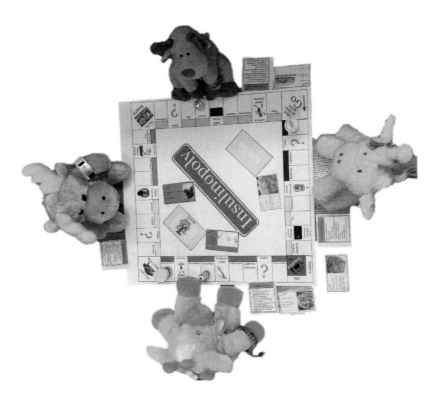

Sometimes we need help
   to learn a little bit
about insulin and food
   to keep me strong and fit.

We have meetings to help us live
   with love, advice and care
learning about food, play, school and sleep
   so my parents and I are aware

So much to learn and do
   Insulin, carbs and tests
They'll help us stay in range
   To keep us at our best

I play with my t1 friends
   While my parents are taught
About diabetes, food and living
   Answers to questions are sought

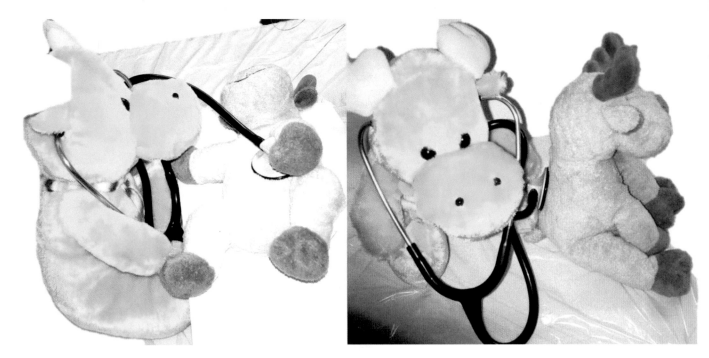

I go to the doc
A couple times a year
He listens to my heart
And looks into my ear.

He listens to my back
And then turns off the light
And looks into my eyes,
As if it were at night.

He checks me out to see
If I'm well and strong,
And that I understand
That I've done nothing wrong.

He asks me what I eat,
At home and school and play.
Checks ears and nose and mouth
To see if I'm okay.

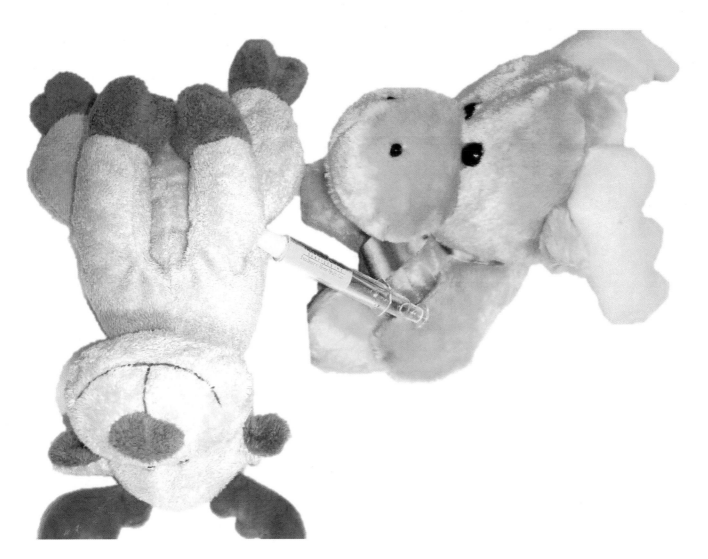

Then he takes my pulse.
   A quick blood test for me
To check what's in my blood
   And find my A1C.

My A1C will tell,
   Has my control been fine?
For the last three months
   Did my sugars climb?

He may ask me to walk
   Or question me to see
Whether I have learned
   To take good care of me.

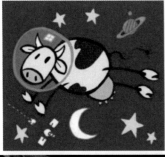
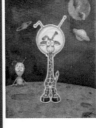
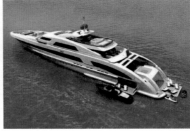
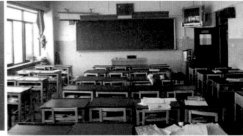

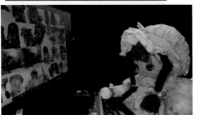

I have diabetes
   But it won't stop me.
I can go in space
   Or sail upon the sea.

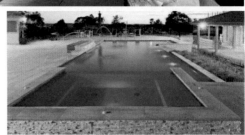

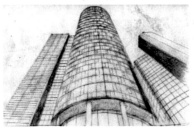

I can fly a plane
   Or I can teach in school.
Computers I can use
   Or swim in a big pool.

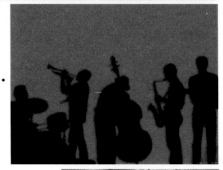

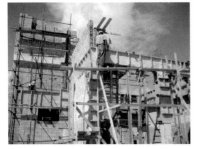

Large buildings I'll design
   And build them well by hand.
Write songs and sing them too,
   Or play in a jazz band.

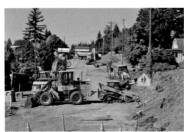

I can run for Senate,
   Or work inside my house.
Feed creatures in the zoo
   Or find a perfect spouse.

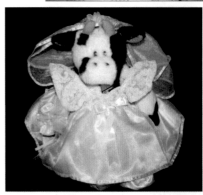

I may work as a chef
   And make great things to eat.
I may work to construct
   A wide and brand-new street.

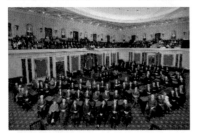

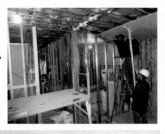

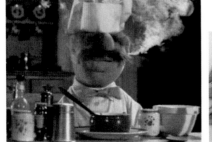
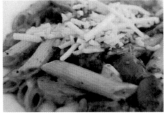
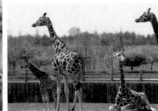
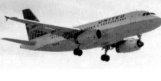

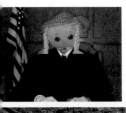
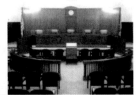
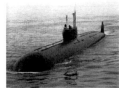
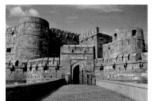
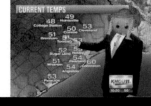

I can be a judge for a case
    Or a lawyer in the court
I can navigate a sub
    Or defend a large fort

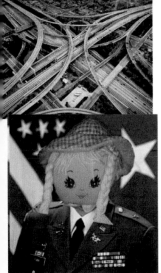
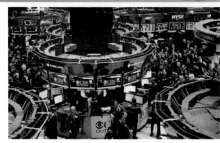

I can be a general,
    Or drive food in a truck
I can predict the weather
    Or design roads that won't get stuck

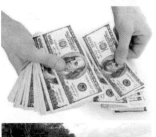
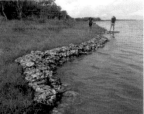

I can make investments that will grow
    Or count money, bonds and stocks
Be a coastal Scientist
    Or a police officer that rocks

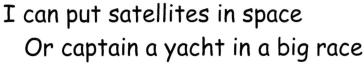

I can build a large windmill
    Or put solar panels still
I can put satellites in space
    Or captain a yacht in a big race

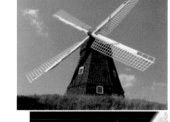
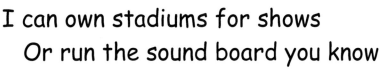
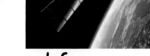

I can own stadiums for shows
    Or run the sound board you know
A rock star performer with guitar
    Or opening up for their acts near and far

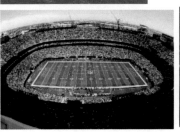
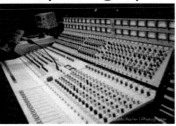
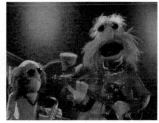
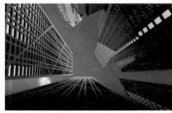

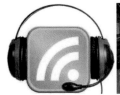
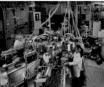
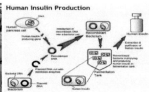
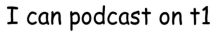
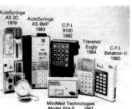
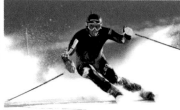

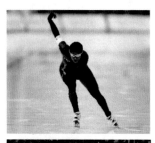

I can podcast on t1
  Or be a research scientist, such fun
I can manufacturer insulin
 Or produce insulin pumps thin

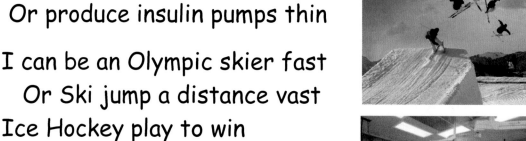

I can be an Olympic skier fast
  Or Ski jump a distance vast
Ice Hockey play to win
  Or speed skate and get a pin

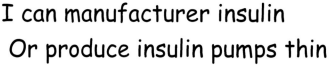

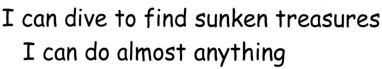

I can teach doctors to operate
  Or cook dinners for the king
I can dive to find sunken treasures
  I can do almost anything

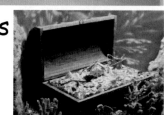

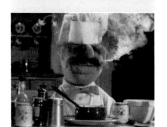

I can design a building tall
  Or lay the foundation so it won't fall
I can write books on giraffes
  Or teach people a new craft

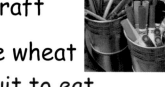

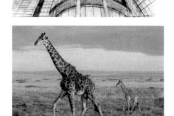

I can farm and grow whole wheat
  Grow vegetables and fruit to eat
I can stock grocery store shelves to sell
  Or if you need water dig a well

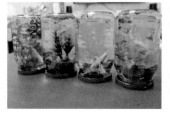

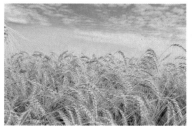
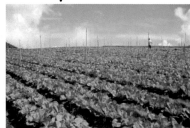
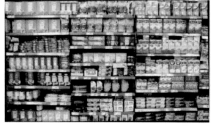
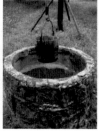

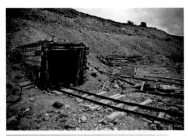
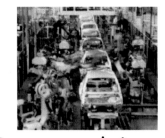
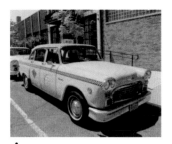
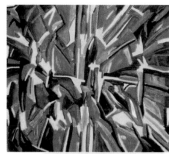
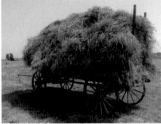
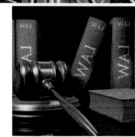

I may work in a mine
   Or factory for cars.
 Might learn to drive a cab
   Take people near and far.

I can paint works of art
   Or drive a big hay cart
I can write laws and get them passed.
   Or blow up buildings with a blast.

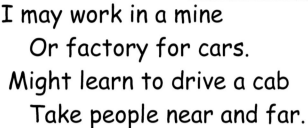
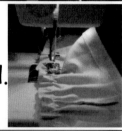
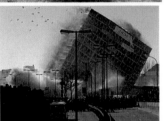

I can sew new clothes
   So that they look great.
 I can paint your walls.
   I bet you cannot wait!

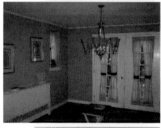
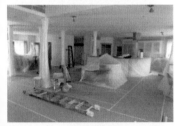
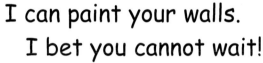
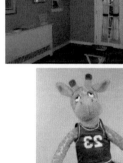

I can host a show
   Or play basketball.
Or drive a fast race car
   Or answer fire calls.

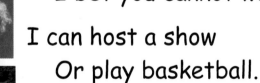
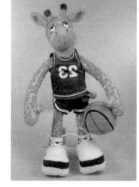

Many of these things
   I may one day do
Don't let diabetes
   Say what you can't do!

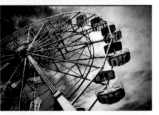
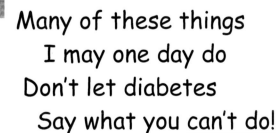
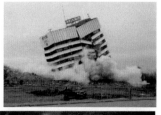
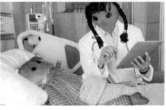
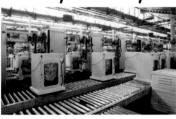
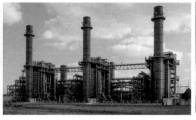
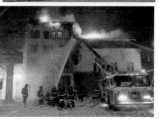

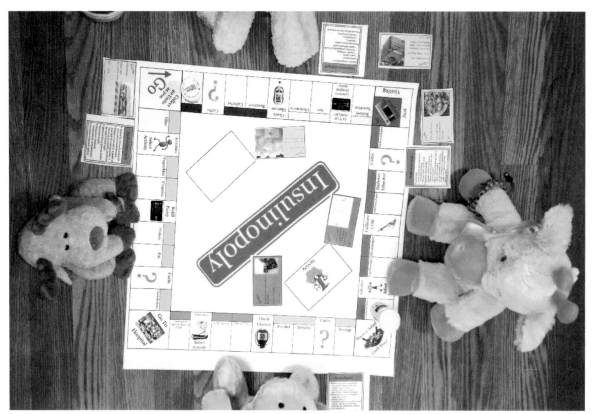

I hope this little book
   Has helped you learn a bit
Of insulin and food
   To keep you strong and fit.

So you'll help others too,
   And show them how it's done.
They may not like the shots
   Or tests, no, they're not fun.

But those things let us live
   A much more healthy life
Taking care with food
   Will keep away the strife.

So much to learn and do.
   Insulin, carbs and tests,
They'll help us stay in range
   To keep us at our best.

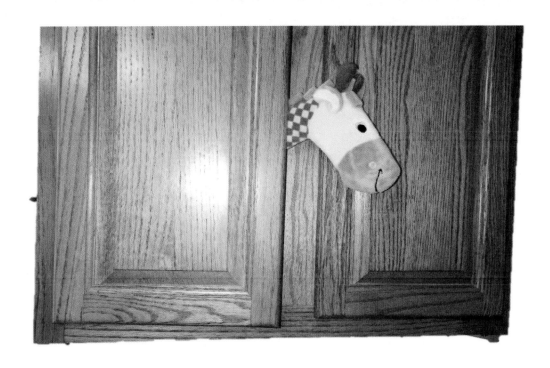

Acknowledgements

To write this book's been fun
   And to all who helped me cope,
I want to give my thanks
   For never losing hope.

My parents didn't know
   If I would survive.
Life was sure not easy then:
   Thank HaShem[1] I'm still alive.

My folks' friends helped me through
   With love, advice and care.
They cooked food just for me
   And I was unaware.

---

[1] G-d

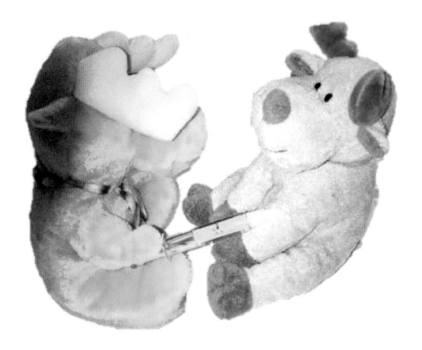

Harry Elias helped
   To clean up all the mess.
Dr. Neustein worked things out,
   These men, HaShem should bless!

Siblings cared for me
   When there was a need.
I hope they read this book
   And enjoy this people seed.

Chula Ruchel gave me shots
   When she was six years old.
Again when I was blind,
   Which helped; she was so bold!

In the dorm Lee Drake
   Saved me from a bus
That really wasn't there.
   Ketones made me fuss!

Mordechai Luria found
  Me dazed and unaware.
He made sure I ate
  And covered every care.

Rav Paltiel, Rabbi Shem Tov
  And all who loved and cared.
Natalie Sera and Sharon Hecht
  Proofread and edited and shared.

Doctors, nurses, techs,
  Family and friend:
Each one had a hand
  Given without end.

All who helped me through
  Wife, Sara Chana, most!
Thanks for your constant help
  Without you I'd be toast!

Said the Rebbe, when I went blind,
  "You won't need laser light.
Your doctors won't believe:
  HaShem has fixed it right!

They only believe in meds
  But teach them as you should.
When adversity seems strong,
  'Think good: it _WILL_ be good!'"

HaShem I thank for all the good.
  Keeping me healthy, alive and at play.
Yerachmiel Altman is my name
  And I thank HaShem each day

Glossary of diabetes-related terms

A full list of diabetes-related terms and their definition can be found on the following web sites among others:
http://www.diabetes.org/diabetes-basics/common-terms/
http://www.everydayhealth.com/diabetes/glossary-of-diabetes-terms.aspx
http://www.webmd.com/diabetes/guide/diabetes-glossary-terms
I have only included those terms which I've used in the book and/or should be a part of everyone's vocabulary.

Acetone: A chemical formed in the blood when the body breaks down fat instead of sugar for energy; if acetone forms, it usually means the cells are starved. Commonly, the body's production of acetone is known as "ketosis." It occurs when there is an absolute or relative deficiency in insulin so sugars cannot get into cells for energy. The body then tries to use other energy sources like proteins from muscle and fat from fat cells. Acetone passes through the body into the urine.

Acidosis: Too much acid in the body, usually from the production of ketones like acetone, when cells are starved; for a person with diabetes, the most common type of acidosis is called "ketoacidosis."

Analog insulin: an altered form of insulin, different from any occurring in nature, but still available to the human body for performing the same action as human insulin in terms of glycemic control. Through genetic engineering of the underlying DNA, the amino acid sequence of insulin can be changed to alter its ADME (absorption, distribution, metabolism, and excretion) characteristics. These modifications have been used to create two types of insulin analogs: those that are more readily absorbed from the injection site and therefore act faster than natural insulin injected subcutaneously, intended to supply the bolus level of insulin needed at mealtime (prandial insulin); and those that are released slowly over a period of between 8 and 24 hours, intended to supply the basal level of insulin during the day and particularly at nighttime (basal insulin).

Basal rate: The amount of insulin required to manage normal daily blood glucose fluctuations; most people constantly produce insulin to manage the glucose fluctuations that occur during the day. In a person with diabetes, giving a constant low level amount of insulin via insulin pump mimics this normal phenomenon.

Blood glucose monitoring or testing: A method of testing how much sugar is in your blood; home blood-glucose monitoring involves pricking your finger with a lancing device, putting a drop of blood on a test strip and inserting the test strip into a blood-glucose-testing meter that displays your blood glucose level. Blood-sugar testing can also be done in the laboratory. Blood-glucose monitoring is recommended three or four times a day for people with insulin-dependent diabetes. Depending on the situation, glucose checks before meals, two hours after meals, at bedtime, in the middle of the night, and before and after exercise may be recommended.

Carbohydrate: One of the three main classes of foods and a source of energy; carbohydrates are mainly sugars and starches that the body breaks down into glucose (a simple sugar that the body can use to feed its cells).

Diabetic ketoacidosis (DKA): A severe, life-threatening condition that results from hyperglycemia (high blood sugar), dehydration, and acid buildup that needs emergency fluid and insulin treatment; DKA happens when there is not enough insulin and cells become starved for sugars. An alternative source of energy called ketones becomes activated. The system creates a buildup of acids. Ketoacidosis can lead to coma and even death.

Emergency medical identification: Cards, bracelets, or necklaces with a written message, used by people with diabetes or other medical problems to alert others in case of a medical emergency, such as coma.

Endocrinologist: A doctor who treats people with hormone problems.

Fasting plasma glucose test (FPG): The preferred method of screening for diabetes; the FPG measures a person's blood sugar level after fasting or not eating anything for at least 8 hours. Normal fasting blood glucose is less than 100 milligrams per deciliter or mg/dL. A fasting plasma glucose greater than 100 mg/dL and less than 126 mg/dL implies that the person has an impaired fasting glucose level but may not have diabetes. A diagnosis of diabetes is made when the fasting blood glucose is greater than 126 mg/dL and when blood tests confirm abnormal results. These tests can be repeated on a subsequent day or by measuring glucose 2 hours after a meal. The results should show an elevated blood glucose of more than 200 mg/dL.

Glucagon: A hormone that raises the level of glucose in the blood by releasing stored glucose from the liver; glucagon is sometimes injected when a person has lost consciousness (passed out) from low blood sugar levels. The injected glucagon helps raise the level of glucose in the blood.

Glucose: A simple sugar found in the blood; it is the body's main source of energy; also known as "dextrose."

Glycated hemoglobin test (HbA1c): This is an important blood test to determine how well you are managing your diabetes; hemoglobin is a substance in red <u>blood cells</u> that carries oxygen to tissues. It can also attach to sugar in the blood, forming a substance called glycated hemoglobin or a <u>Hemoglobin A1C</u>. The test provides an average blood sugar measurement over a 6- to 12-week period and is used in conjunction with home glucose monitoring to make treatment adjustments. The ideal range for people with diabetes is generally less than 7%. This test can also be used to diagnose diabetes when the HbA1c level is equal to or greater than 6.5%.

Human insulin: Bio-engineered insulin very similar to insulin made by the body; the DNA code for making human insulin is put into bacteria or yeast cells and the insulin made is purified and sold as human insulin.

Hyperglycemia: High blood sugar; this condition is fairly common in people with diabetes. Many things can cause hyperglycemia. It occurs when the body does not have enough insulin or cannot use the insulin it does have.

Insulin: A hormone produced by the pancreas that helps the body use sugar for energy; the beta cells of the pancreas make insulin.

Insulin pump: A small, computerized device – about the size of a small cell phone – that is worn on a belt or put in a pocket; insulin pumps have a small flexible tube with a fine needle on the end. The needle is inserted under the skin of the abdomen and taped in place. A carefully measured, steady flow of insulin is released into the body.

Insulin reaction: Another term for hypoglycemia in a person with diabetes; this occurs when a person with diabetes has injected too much insulin, eaten too little food, or exercised without eating extra food.

Insulin shock: A severe condition that occurs when the level of blood sugar drops quickly.

Ketone bodies: Often simply called ketones, one of the products of fat burning in the body; when there is not enough insulin, your body is unable to use sugar (glucose) for energy and your body breaks down its own fat and protein. When fat is used, ketone bodies, an acid, appear in your urine and blood. A large amount of ketones in your system can lead to a serious condition called ketoacidosis. Ketones can be detected and monitored in your urine at home using products such as <u>Ketostix</u>, <u>Chemstrips</u>, and Acetest. When your blood sugar is consistently greater than 250 mg/dl, if you are ill or pregnant and have diabetes, ketones should be checked regularly.

Lancet: A fine, sharp-pointed needle for pricking the skin; used in blood sugar monitoring.

Podiatrist: A health professional who diagnoses and treats <u>foot problems</u>.

Rapid-acting Insulin: Covers insulin needs for meals eaten at the same time as the injection; this type of insulin is used with longer-acting insulin. Includes <u>Humalog</u>, <u>Novolog</u>, and <u>Apidra</u>.

Self-blood glucose monitoring: Performed at home; see blood glucose monitoring or testing.

Type 1 diabetes: A type of diabetes in which the insulin-producing cells (called beta cells) of the pancreas are damaged; people with type 1 diabetes produce little or no insulin, so glucose cannot get into the body's cells for use as energy. This causes blood sugar to rise. People with type 1 diabetes must use insulin injections to control their blood sugar.

Type 2 diabetes: A type of diabetes in which the insulin produced is either not enough or the person's body does not respond normally to the amount present; therefore, glucose in the blood cannot get into the body's cells for use as energy. This results in an increase in the level of glucose (sugar) in the blood.

Organizations for further information

American Association of Diabetes Educators https://www.diabeteseducator.org

American Diabetes Association (ADA) http://www.diabetes.org/?loc=logo

Beyond Type 1 https://beyondtype1.org/

Center for Disease Control (CDC) http://www.cdc.gov/diabetes/home/index.html

Children with Diabetes (CWD) http://www.childrenwithdiabetes.com/

Diabetes Research Institute https://www.diabetesresearch.org/

Insulin Pumpers http://www.insulin-pumpers.org/

Insulinopoly https://www.facebook.com/groups/Insulinopoly/

Jewish Friends With Diabetes International www.friendswithdiabetes.org

Juvenile Diabetes Research Foundation (JDRF) http://jdrf.org/

Medic Alert Foundation http://www.medicalert.org/

Medline Plus – Diabetes in Children and Teens
  https://medlineplus.gov/diabetesinchildrenandteens.html

National Association of School Nurses https://www.nasn.org

National Institute of Diabetes and Digestive and Kidney Diseases
  https://www.niddk.nih.gov/health-information/diabetes

National Institute of Health - Medline – Diabetes (NIH)
  https://medlineplus.gov/diabetes.html

NeedyMeds (*Find help with the cost of medicine*)
  http://www.needymeds.org/drp.taf?filename=diabetes.htm

Parenting Diabetic Kids http://www.parentingdiabetickids.com/

PubMed Diabetes https://www.ncbi.nlm.nih.gov/pubmed/?term=Diabetes

SafeNeedleDisposal.org https://safeneedledisposal.org

T1International https://www.t1international.com/

Companies which provide tools and help

A Silly Patch	https://asillypatch.com/
Dexcom	http://www.dexcom.com/
Fifty50 Medical	https://www.fifty50pharmacy.com/
Frio: Insulin Cooling Case	http://frioinsulincoolingcase.com/
Grandma's Hands	http://www.grandmashands.ca/
GrifGrips	https://www.grifgrips.com/
Medic Alert Foundation	http://www.medicalert.org/
Medicool health & beauty	http://medicool.com/diabetes/
Medtronic Diabetes	http://www.medtronicdiabetes.com/home
Myabetic	https://www.myabetic.com/
Pump Innerwear	https://www.pocketinnerwear.com/
Pump Wear	https://www.pumpwearinc.com/
Pump Peelz	https://pumppeelz.com/
Road iD	https://www.roadid.com/
Tallygear	http://www.tallygear.com/
Tandem Diabetes	https://www.tandemdiabetes.com/
Tidepool	https://tidepool.org/
Unomedical	http://www.infusion-set.com/
Wearing Dabbee	http://wearingdabbee.com/en/

I can help take care of me ²ⁿᵈ ᵉᵈⁱᵗⁱᵒⁿ

Learning to Live with Diabetes for Children
Book Series (3 Books)

Endorsements

"*I can help take care of me*" by Yerachmiel Altman is a touching and poignant journey through the past and present world of type 1 diabetes as voiced by from the author's inner child.... Altman seeks to both inspire and entertain us through his poetic narrative. I strongly recommend parents of children with diabetes reading this book to their d-children. It will be time WELL spent.

Stephen W. Ponder, MD, FAAP, CDE
Author of Sugar Surfing

"*I can help take care of Me*" is a charming and creative book which helps children and their families learn about type 1 diabetes.

The basics of diabetes treatment are illustrated. Insulin syringes, blood sugar testing, sugar testing devices (glucometers), insulin pumps and continuous glucose monitors are utilized by the adorable stuffed animal.

Stephanie B. Brett-Bell, LICSW, ACSW

I Can Help Take Care of Me is an educational story about Diabetes (Type 1) written by Yerachmiel B. Altman. This illustrated children's book, written completely in rhyming poetry and using soft toys as patient, parent and doctor.

When your symptoms alert you to the fact that something is not right, it is essential that your blood sugar and blood pressure are checked and that your blood sugar is brought back to the proper range before you can partake in sports or play with your friends. The book makes it very clear that Diabetes is not contagious in any way, and that when you eat well and take proper care of yourself, there is absolutely nothing that stops you from being able to live a full and happy life.

As a Diabetic, I was quite impressed with how Yerachmiel B. Altman tackled such a difficult topic, especially for children, who can be quite upset, angry and stubborn when diagnosed with Diabetes. The earlier they are educated on all aspects of the disease and are taught that Diabetes is not a death sentence, the better. When a Diabetic child realizes how important it is to tell the people around them that they are not feeling well, it soon becomes second nature to them to take care of themselves and to alert others that they may be in danger. Yerachmiel B. Altman has not only taken the mystery, stigma and fear out of Diabetes, but has also taught a child to feel empowered, in that they are more aware of their symptoms than anybody else and can play a part in making sure they are well. Educating parents about the fact that their children cannot catch the disease from those with Diabetes is also covered. I recommend I Can Help Take Care of Me to all newly diagnosed Diabetics, their friends, families, and peers.

Reviewed By Rosie Malezer for Readers' Favorite

Made in the USA
San Bernardino, CA
24 June 2020

74070836R00038